MW01107988

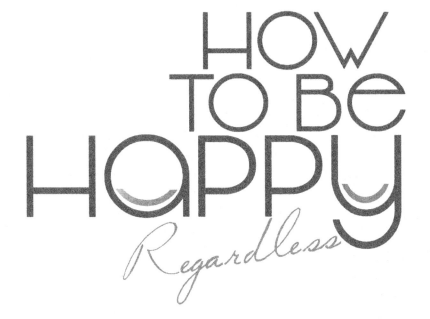

HOW TO BE HAPPY

Regardless

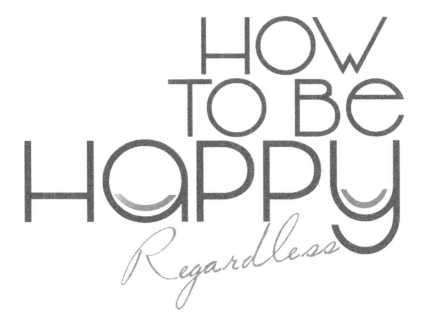

james e. woods

Table of Contents

One   Choose To Be Happy   9

Two   Cultivate Thanksgiving   12
         The second step to becoming happy

Three   Practice Forgiveness   15
         Step three to becoming happy

Four   Counteract Thoughts and Feelings   18
         Step four to becoming happy
         The Key to Thoughts

Five   Money Will Not Make You Happy   22
         Step five to becoming happy
         What is money?

Six   Foster Friendships   25
         Step six to becoming happy

Seven   Engage in Worthwhile Activities   28

Eight   Health Issues   31

Nine   Divorce   35

Ten   Grief   38

Eleven   Suicide   42

Twelve   The End and The Beginning   46

Foreword

Dr. James E. Woods, II, scholar and teacher, eloquently combines his anointed words with practical lessons in simplicity. Every work, but especially this volume, is no exception. This manual can help any serious believer to rise above personal circumstances to the place of victory that Jesus intended.

Following the several steps enumerated by Dr. Woods, every reader can rise above the weak and beggarly elements of life. Happiness becomes a reality in this book designed to help the helpless. Drawing from personal experience and common sense from the Word of God, this Pastor shares easily implemented steps to remedy current situations and prevent other ones.

This is not a quick fix, 12-step plan to temporary relief, but rather a long-term permanent deliverance based on the Truth.

The text is accompanied by a workbook geared to each chapter of the book, reinforcing important points to guarantee the readers' success in life. I highly recommend Dr. Woods' writings, this one and his other books available on Amazon.

Dr. Patricia L. Powell

Introduction

For most people happiness occurs when a set of ideal circumstances fall into place. This type of happiness is illusory and subject to external forces beyond the average person's control. Happiness based on external factors that change from moment to moment produce a rollercoaster of emotions. In How To Be Happy Regardless you will learn how to take charge of your life by releasing internal forces as a shield of protection from the ever-changing situations of daily living.

Regardless means in spite of or without concern. The purpose of this book is to learn to be happy in spite of circumstances. For every reason to be unhappy there are an equal, and in many cases, greater and other reasons to be happy. Being Happy Regardless requires a redirection of focus toward the things that facilitate happiness while simultaneously deemphasizing the influence of circumstances that lead toward your unhappiness.

This book contains a blueprint, and when followed, could produce change. Being happy doesn't mean the absence of problems, but rather the ability to manage how well you deal with and work your way through problems. By following the instructions outlined in this book happiness will become a vibrant force for day-to-day living, regardless.

one
Choose To Be Happy

"There is only one cause of unhappiness: the false beliefs you have in your head, beliefs so widespread, so commonly held, that it never occurs to you to question them."
—Anthony de Mello

It was the worst of time and the worst of time. After a period in which I witnessed the death of a family member, two very close friends, a series of personal health issues, and the loss of $72,000.00 a year in income, I found myself going from pastoring approximately one thousand people to only eleven people, in less than two years. Everyone has a list of things they believe makes them happy. Here was my list at the time: Family, friends, income, occupational success, and health. All of these were changed or gone in a two-year period.

What was I to do? How was I to go on? I was overwhelmed. Making matters worse, I internalized everything. I felt there was no one in whom to confide. So, I lingered in my unhappiness. Ironically, when in the company of others, I put on a happy face. Inside I was hurting.

The most difficult times came when no one was around. Whenever I was alone, most of my time was spent rehearsing my situation. I did not think I was feeling sorry for myself. I just thought things were bad.

As it turned out, my thinking was the biggest part of my problem. The more I thought about my situation, the more it, my thoughts, overwhelmed me. I started paying attention to how much of my time was spent thinking about my unhappiness. This led me to a conclusion: I had to decide to be happy, regardless. Without that decision nothing would change.

Each day I reinforced my decision to be happy, regardless. At first, nothing seemed to change. As a matter of fact, some things got worst. However, I stood my ground. Bit by bit change in the right direction began. I first noticed it in my thinking, and then my mood. Before long other areas improved. This book, in part, presents the things I learned on the way to being happy, regardless.

I will begin with the first thing you must do on your way to personal happiness. You must choose to be happy. Choosing to be happy will not get your old job back, will not reverse the divorce decree, and will not put the money back in your account. Choosing to be happy is about changing and empowering YOU. The power to choose to be happy cannot be taxed by the IRS, repo-ed by a creditor, or divided up in a divorce. It is yours free and clear. You can choose to be happy anywhere, in the hospital or the prison. You can exercise this choice at home, work, or in court.

Choosing to be happy is simple but not always easy. The difficulty is rooted in the feelings that feed our unhappiness. These feelings have to be overridden. There is only one way to do this, and that is with AC-TION. The first and most important action for you to begin your journey is to take control of the words you speak.

What to say and what not to say

It is important to know what to say as well as what not to say. People underestimate both the value and influence of words. But science is learning more every day about how our words affect feelings, attitude, and even our health. The first action you need to take after you choose to be happy is to give voice to that choice. This is done by declaring your intentions to be happy.

How you feel about doing this is irrelevant. Your feelings are what you are fighting to change. So, do not listen to them as they battle with you for control. Your feelings will want you to say the things you should not say. Feelings will remind you of all the things you do not have, and therefore, feelings will want you to inventory all of your lack. That is contrary to your choice to be happy.

Start each day with an affirmation of your choice to be happy. It can be as simple as, "I choose to be happy." Or, "Today I want to be happy regardless of how I feel." Develop whatever phrasing works best for you. There are dozens of books on affirmations. These books are available in both religious and secular forms.

I would like to end this chapter with a promise and a warning. If you commit to making the choice to be happy, it will be the first step to turning your life around. It will empower you to regain the control that is rightfully yours. Choosing to be happy is not a magic pill. Many of the problems you are facing will still be there. But by choosing to be happy, you will begin to transform yourself into the person who is capable of overcoming these problems. However, if you do not commit to and stick with this first step the rest of this book will be of very little use to you. You may very well be prolonging the time spent away from the happiness to which you are entitled.

One final note, I have known the joys of happiness and the despair of being unhappy. Being happy is much better. I find it interesting that the Bible uses a different word for happy. It refers to the happy person as "Blessed". When you choose to be happy, it is a choice to be blessed.

You are about to make a choice that could lead to the blessed life. Why would you put it off another day?

two
Cultivate Thanksgiving

Bible commentator Matthew Henry, after being robbed, wrote in his diary the following: "Let me be thankful. First, because I was never robbed before. Second, because although they took my wallet, they did not take my life. Third, because although they took my all, it was not much. Fourth, because it was I who was robbed, not I who robbed."

The second step to becoming happy:

The next step in your journey toward happiness is to cultivate or exercise being thankful as a daily routine. No matter how bad things may seem everyone has something for which to be thankful.

It was May 5, 2014; I woke up in the hospital. Once aware of my surroundings I checked to see the results of the surgery. My right leg was gone below the knee. At that moment I had a choice to make: be upset over the loss of the leg, or try to be thankful.

I thought the most obvious thing; I was alive. But being thankful would require more than that. I expanded my view of the situation. Six months before the amputation, it started with a black spot under a toenail and grew into a major infection. I had to sleep sitting up in a chair. Every time I tried to lay down, it felt as though a steel spike was being driven through my foot. Only by having my foot in the down position would the pain leave.

Night after night I sat in the chair doing my best to sleep. During the day things seemed reasonable. But as night time approached I dreaded my nightly ritual. On a good evening, I slept four hours. Good nights were the exception.

My doctors recommended hyperbaric theory. I had gone through the therapy before with great results. But this time, it was of no help at all. The nights turn into weeks and the weeks into months.

One thing I was unaware of was changes in my demeanor and attitude. Being in pain for so long was changing me, and not in a nice way. The pain made me focus on myself with no regard for anyone else. This changing mindset damaged relationships. But the pain blinded me to all of this.

My doctors recommended amputating my big toe; after all, it was the problem. I agreed, anything to relieve the pain. However, the procedure only made things worst. The damage spread to the other toes. Let me take a moment to state: I am not a diabetic. Now the doctors wanted to take half my foot. Half a foot is better than none, so I agreed. Unfortunately, it was not enough to solve the problem. I was still in pain.

That brings me back to May 5, 2014, and being thankful. As I lay on my back in that hospital bed faced with the loss of my leg and needing to find reasons for being thankful, a smile broke out on my face. Yes, I had been in pain for six months, and yes, I had slept in a chair for six months. Yes, I had lost my foot and part of a leg. But I was thankful, not just for being alive; I was thankful because the pain was gone.

Family and friends came to see me. They would enter my room as if coming to a wake only to find me setting up and smiling. I told them how thankful I was to be able to lie down and sleep. Most of my visitors thought something was wrong with me. However, I was truly grateful.

One of the keys to being thankful is being honest regarding what is going right in your life. For example: if you are reading this book you are, you can see. If this book is being read to you, you can hear. If you bought this book, you value your life. If someone gave it to you, rather family, friend, or a total stranger, someone sees value in you.

There are many things life throws our way to distract us from being thankful. It is important not allow these beguilements to stop us. When circumstances, events, or people come between us and being thankful, recognize things for what they are, distractions. At that very moment it is up to us to decide, will we be drawn away from thankfulness or will we fight to maintain the peace of Thanksgiving.

When a car breaks down, a tow truck is summoned. The tow truck hooks up to the stranded vehicle and pulls it to a new location. Thankfulness is our tow truck. It pulls us away from situations that break us down and keep us stuck. Used regularly, thankfulness will prevent us from breaking down on the side of life's road.

Do not wait for a better day, or the right moment; start where you are. Take time out, and consider just how many things you can find to give thanks. It may be difficult in the beginning, but with time you will be thankful for many things presently taken for granted. The reason I am so confident this will work for you is based on brain science. Once you require your brain to focus on a direction, it will continue to reach out in that direction. This process works both ways. Think about what is wrong with your life, and the brain will direct its attention on how many bad things it can locate. All you need to do is redirect your thinking toward being thankful.

three
Practice Forgiveness

A man who was telling his friend about an argument he'd had with his wife commented, "Oh, how I hate it, every time we have an argument; she gets historical."
The friend replied, "You mean hysterical."
"No," he insisted. "I mean historical. Every time we argue she drags up everything from the past and holds it against me!"

Step three to becoming happy:

The next step in becoming happy is to practice forgiveness. Holding onto past hurts can affect physical as well as mental health. The dirty secret about un-forgiveness is that it hurts the one not forgiving far more than the un-forgiven.

As a Christian, I am expected to forgive no matter what others do. Years ago I was hired to solve a major problem for a large non-profit organization. We had an agreement, and the date was set. Because of the job's location, it was in my family's best interest if we relocated. So, I packed up the wife and children, and we moved.

The organization's biggest problem was a leadership vacuum. When I arrived the group was facing a fifty-percent drop in donations. They were spending two thousand dollars more a week than what was coming in. Savings were almost gone, morale was at an all-time low, and quality staffers were leaving. The organization was eighteen months from closing its doors. The remaining leadership expected me to turn things around, and for the money they paid, the leadership was well within their rights.

In six months income was up to its highest levels ever, expenses were down, and morale was up. All indicators were well in the green, and the books were in the black. While I am ashamed to admit it, I expected a parade in my honor.

What they gave me was a nice letter informing me that my services were no longer needed. I was fired. At first I was shocked, then angry, and finally, hurt. Apparently, I performed as expected; the organization was back on top. The staff was impressed with the turnaround. Key people had returned, and new people added. But I was still fired.

I am a professional, and as such, it was important that I exercise decorum, i.e. do not make trouble. Like a good soldier I conducted myself accordingly. Inwardly was a different matter; I spent the next ten years unwilling to forgive those people for what they had done. Also, I also could not forgive myself for taking the job and putting my family through that situation.

The day finally came when I ran into one of the individuals that signed my letter of separation. He greeted me as though nothing had ever happened! I could not believe him; he was smiling and everything. Not wanting to be outdone, I smiled back.

After this encounter was over, I was faced with an uncomfortable truth: I wasted ten years angry, bitter and unwilling to forgive, while the people who had done this to me went on with their lives. Although I was stuck in the past, they had moved on into the future.

William Shakespeare's character, Prospero, when finally given a chance to punish those who had removed him from his rightful place as king, states, "Let us not burden our remembrance with a heaviness that's gone." ("The Tempest")

That is what I had done, burdened my remembrance. When we hold onto past hurts and will not forgive the people involved or ourselves, we are the ones carrying the weight. The longer we keep the weight, the heavier it gets. It becomes too much, and we become bitter. By forgiving, the power of bad events to create bitterness and resentment is reduced. Let it go. It's too heavy.

There is another aspect of forgiveness that no honest effort to address the subject can omit. That is the forgiveness that comes from God.

Why Wilson Was Hanged

In 1829 George Wilson, in Pennsylvania, was sentenced by a United States Court for robbing the mail and for murder. President Andrew Jackson pardoned him, but this was refused. Wilson insisted that it was not a pardon unless he accepted it. That was a point of law never before raised, and the President called upon the Supreme Court to decide.

Chief Justice John Marshall gave the following decision: "A pardon is a paper, the value of which depends upon its acceptance by the person implicated. It is hardly to be supposed that one under sentence of death would refuse to accept a pardon, but if it is refused, it is no pardon. George Wilson must be hanged!" And he was hanged.

Provisionally the gospel of Christ which is the power of God unto salvation is for everyone irrespective of what he may be or what he may have done. Potentially, it is only to "everyone that believeth."
--Sunday School Times

If you would embrace the forgiveness that God offers, He will empower you to extend to others the forgiveness you have received. Like choosing to be happy, or thankful, again the power to forgive is up to you. But if you ever hope to know true happiness, forgiveness is not optional.

four
Counteract Thoughts and Feelings

What Do You Think About?

Ralph Waldo Emerson was correct in asserting, "Man is what he thinks about all day long." That which he or she feeds on, the context of his/her experience, the playbacks from previous contacts, all have frightening and sometimes wonderful means of shaping and strengthening life.

Step four to becoming happy:

The next step on the road to being happy is to take control of your thoughts. You can learn to recognize and challenge thoughts you have about being inadequate and helpless. By gaining control of this area of your life, it will change everything.

Thoughts are like automobiles, big and powerful. Cars are much stronger than the people who drive them. But a car will not go anywhere without fuel and a driver. Thoughts are the same way; they require fuel and a driver to go anywhere. This truth is the key to gaining control over negative thoughts. Deny negative thoughts by replacing these ideas with other thoughts.

The Key to Thoughts:

Thoughts are driven by focus. By changing your focus, you can change your mind. A classic example is when a person is getting an injection. Needles hurt, but if you look away and focus on something else the pain is lessened. Why? Because you changed your thinking by changing your focus. But if you think about how much that injection will hurt it hurts a lot. Take someone whose focus is on their divorce. All day they will focus on the relationship that is no more, thinking and dealing with feelings of rejection and betrayal. At every opportunity, they rehearse what was done to them. Do not misunderstand me; divorce can be painful. But like getting a needle, by changing your focus, you will lessen the pain.

There are two primary ways to change your focus. One way to change or redirect your focus is to change what you are seeing. Stop looking at pictures of people who have hurt you. Do not read their text messages or watch movies you once enjoyed together. Forgetting your ex can be a big challenge for mothers who have to look at their children and see the father. But you know that their father is not the only thing you see when you look at them. They are your kids; focus on things about them rather than who they resemble.

The second of two primary ways to change your focus is to change what you are listening to. The Bible says, "...Faith comes by hearing..." Make every effort to listen to things that shift your focus in positive directions. The right music, motivational talks, and uplifting sermons can do wonders for your focus. I recommend you spend one hour a day listening to something that drives your concentration in the right direction.

Feelings: "The battle you are going through is not fueled by words or actions of others; it is fueled by the mind that gives it importance"
– Shannon L. Alder

Feelings, unlike thoughts, can be affected by many things. But like thoughts, there are a few things you can do to override negative feelings. Most people do not realize the connection between thoughts and feelings. Like thoughts, feelings need fuel to run on. Unlike thoughts, feelings do not require fuel to get started. This is why people can have feelings with no basis in reality.

You do not need a doctorate in human behavior to know that humans were never designed to live primarily by their feelings. While they have a place, feelings serve to add dimension to our humanity, not to control it. There are many positive things that can come from feelings, but left unchecked those same feelings can destroy families, ruin finances, and bring nations to war. Feelings, like children, need boundaries. A child will run into the street with no regard for the consequences. Feelings can lead people into relationships or situations again with no regard for the consequences.

The truth about feelings is that they can lie to you. You read that correctly; your feelings can lie to you. They can convince you of things that have no basis in reality. Many beautiful people have allowed feelings to put them in despair, battling daily feelings of inadequacy and helplessness. What is the foundation of these beliefs? Before you answer that question, understand that your feelings never deal with facts. Just because your ex-spouse told you that you were a worthless person has no real basis for you to feel empty. If your ex called you a banana, would you to feel like one? Why not? Because you would override their statement with reality. Just remember: it was your feelings that told you how wonderful your ex was.

Two keys to taking control of negative emotions would be: One, judge your feelings with reality. Ask yourself "Regardless of how I feel, what is the truth that sees beyond this feeling? I am not asking you to ignore the fact that you are hurting. I am asking you to look beyond today's pain to a better tomorrow. The facts will help you see things for what they are. Rejection is a difficult feeling to overcome, but with the correct application of the facts, you can make it.

The second way to take control of feelings is with actions. Negative attitude seeks to immobilize. These feelings make you want to stay in the house, quit your job, stick your head in the sand. When you chose action regardless of how you feel, you will discover a powerful truth. Feelings follow actions! Start acting better and you will soon start feeling better. Acting makes the brain function accordingly. Force moves in a positive direction, and the brain will start working to bring everything in line with that direction, your thoughts, and feelings.

Focus to control your thoughts. Act to control your feelings.

five

Money Will Not Make You Happy

*Money cannot buy peace of mind. It cannot heal ruptured relation-
ships, or build meaning into a life that has none.*

— Richard M. De Vos, Billionaire

Step five to becoming happy:

What is money?

Anything of value that serves as a (1) generally accepted medium of
financial exchange, (2) legal tender for repayment of debt, (3) standard
of value, (4) unit of accounting measure, and (5) means to save or store
purchasing power. *(The Business Dictionary.com)*

Why is there this assumption that money, or enough money will produce happiness?

The first thing you should notice is that the word "happy" is not men-
tioned in the definition. Money is a tool. Like all tools, money's effec-
tiveness rests not in money itself, but in the skill level of the one using it.
But even with the greatest of money skills it still lacks the power to make
you happy.

Tools multiply effort. A saw increases the amount of wood you can cut in a given time frame, as opposed to cutting it with a butter knife. An electric saw, a better tool, will multiply the same effort more. The same tools use improperly can cause significant harm.

As with all tools, you can use them regardless of whether or not you are happy. If money were a happy pill, just some of it should produce some happiness. Interviews held with lottery winners have shown that the money did not produce the desired effect. Because they had lived under the illusion that money would make them happy, when the reality of money's impotence in that area was realized, they became anything but happy.

At the heart of why people believe money will make them happy is the things they can do with money: Get out of debt, buy new things, move to a better home, live an all-around better lifestyle. The flaw in this is the assumption that the bills, the lack of things, their current house or lifestyle is why they are unhappy. But as we learned in chapter one, you have to choose to be happy. And if you do not have money now, learn to be happy before you get some.

Why should you learn to be happy apart from money?

As stated before money is a tool, and as such it multiplies or amplifies effort. Herein is the danger: money will increase the state for which it is used. If you are unhappy with the money, when it comes, it will multiply or amplify your situation by empowering you to act on a larger scale. For instance, people are surprised to read about the athlete who signs a multi-million-dollar contract, only to be caught and arrested with tens of thousands of dollars' worth of drugs. The money did not make him happy. It just multiplied the number of narcotics, the degree of his unhappiness, and what he could buy.

Let me be clear: Money does pay bills which could take some pressure off of you. Money can help you acquire things, which could make some aspects of your life easier. But happiness is not the absence of bills or a new house. Some of the things you will use the money for will bring on new issues.

In my lifetime I have met and spoken to several millionaires. Without exception, they all in one form or another were very clear that money was just a tool. Money cannot bring meaning into life; it can only work with what is there.

What has money done for you lately?

One of the last big things I spent money on was a vacation. My wife and I had a great time. It was an exciting time. But excitement is not happiness. If we were not happy before the trip, spending the money on the vacation would not have produced happiness.

If people were honest, they would admit to having had money, but it was never enough. Because once gone you are confronted with the truth; the money did not make you happy. Money can no more make you happy than a screwdriver can make you happy. Now, if you need a screwdriver, you will be glad to have one, but that is not happiness.

The fifth step toward being happy is realizing the proper place of money as a tool, not the means of acquiring happiness. There is nothing wrong with wanting to earn more money. Just do not con yourself into believing your lack of happiness is a money issue. Many people find themselves in jobs they hate, but not because the job is so bad. Remember how excited you were when you got that job, but stopped choosing to be happy about the job. Amazingly, if that job ended tomorrow, they would spend the next five years telling everyone, "What an excellent job I had!"

Finally, if you find yourself deep in debt, you need to stop creating new debt. If money will not make you happy, debt is even less likely. In some cases people are not unhappy because of debt. They created the debt, because they were unhappy. Either way, debt can be an indication of misunderstanding the real function of money. IT IS ONLY A TOOL.

six
Foster Friendships

A man that hath friends must shew himself friendly: and there is a friend that sticketh closer than a brother.

Proverbs 18:24 (KJV)

Step six to becoming happy:

F riendship is a type of relationship between two people who care about each other. This definition is an over-simplification. A friend is the first person you want to call with good news. A friend is a person who puts up with you when you were unreasonable. A friend is a person who says how you look in that outfit.

I was asked to do a presentation for an organization. I did everything possible to prepare for the event. I did proper audience analysis, pre-event site inspection, and other things essential for a successful event presentation.

The day arrived, and I was as ready as I could be. I showed up early and made sure everything was in place. The moment had come; all the planning and preparation was at this time. I was introduced and walked onto the stage. For the next forty-five minutes, the presentation went better than I could have imagined. At the end, I received a standing

25

ovation. I must admit it felt magnificent. But for a brief moment, I had a thought, "The planning and preparations had nothing to do with it. I'm just that good." Yes, I had, lost my mind, but right in the middle of this ego trip, one of my dearest friends came to me and said, "Jim, you are good. But you are not as good as they think you are."

You may think that was a cold thing to say, especially from a friend, but as my friend, he is also the one that helps me deal with reality. He knew that I was not thin-skinned, and could put his comments in perspective.

We as humans are wired to need people in our lives. While family can fill some of that need, there is a part of us that requires volunteer relationships. Individuals are involved in our lives because they chose to be. Several mental illnesses are due to a lack of these connections in people's lives.

One of the significant challenges of long-term space exploration is how to develop a group of individuals who can survive long-term isolation even with a spaceship filled with fellow travelers. Knowing they have traveled away from family and friends will cause emotional breakdowns. Everyone has two great psychological needs: One, is the need to be loved, and the second is the need to love someone. This need is apart from anything sexual. It has its fulfillment in friendships. This need explains why couples who develop a true friendship first stay married longer, because these two people are friends by choice.

Most people want friends, friends who will stick with them, friends who will be there, no matter what comes, and friends who will be helpful in a time of need. Like Proverbs 18:24b says "...closer than a brother."

How can a person have these types of friends? What does it take to attract these friends? The answer may be one of the biggest, and therefore hardest truth for you to face. But it is worth the rewards it will bring you.

The middle portion of the quote says," ...Must show himself friendly..." Before you can rightfully expect to have the type of friends you want, or more importantly need, you must become that kind of friend to others. Herein lays the rub: some laws govern life. One such law is reciprocity. This law, also known as reaping what you sow, works just as sure as gravity. This law drives creation to react to your actions. You cannot stick your head in the sand complaining about the friends you do not have, and simultaneously be unwilling to be friendly and expect things to get better. You are reading this book because you want things to change.

Today you must purpose to be the friend someone else needs. Take your mind off your issues, and focus on someone else. I have learned, if I help people who are dealing with the same problem, while helping them I get the solution needed for my situation.

You have gifts and talents that God has given you, use them to reach out and befriend someone. You be that friend that is closer than a brother. You be the one somebody can lean on. As you show yourself friendly, others, not necessarily the one you are helping, will be real friends to you.

Fostering friendships is the act of doing the things that cause the friendship to grow. One thing that fosters friendships is investing time understanding the hopes and dreams of others, by taking the time to listen to someone when you want to talk about your own business or plans. It also requires you to know how to be helpful, without just being critical.

One of the benefits we derive from friendships is personal growth. Each friend you develop has knowledge, talents, or skills you lack. Your association with them will expose you to insights you would lack without them. Another benefit of friendships is you get to see both your limitations and potential through the eyes of your friends. In short, friends can provoke you to do better and keep you from making a fool of yourself.

If you truly desire to be happy, it is important that you cultivate friendships. Maybe, before you try to start new friendships, you should restore some old ones, if possible.

seven
Engage in Worthwhile Activities

Step seven to becoming happy:

B eing unhappy causes stagnation. Over time, your thinking, and even your physical activities will slow down from their natural flow. Your life will be running in slow motion. This stagnation will spill over into every area of your life. You will develop attitudes toward your job, co-workers, and even your boss. If not stopped this state of being will bring you to complete immobilization.

Once completely immobilized getting out of bed becomes a struggle every day. It can go as far as to cause any chore to be a battle. This fight is the inward side of the conflict. Externally this immobilization will cause you to be antisocial.

You come to a place where you isolate yourself. The sad thing is all your reasons for avoiding people will start to make sense. The longer you avoid people, the easier it gets to continue the practice. There is only one way to break this cycle.

Do not sit around the house feeling sorry for yourself. Get engaged or thoroughly absorbed in a meaningful activity that challenges your abilities. Getting involved will break all three levels of the cycle, stagnation, immobilization, and antisocial behavior. It will take time, but many of the benefits will materialize sooner than you think.

Becoming active will energize you mentally and physically. Replace the thoughts that have you running around in circles with the idea of your new activities. Being involved will drive you out of your bed and into the real world. The habits you formed during your period of immobilization will fade away as new life-affirming activities replace them.

Becoming involved infuses your life with purpose. Instead of wearing people out with invitations to a pity party, you become an advocate for your new found activities. People will want to hear what you have to say because it will be something meaningful.

How do you begin? Find groups that need your skills or talents. Make yourself and what God blessed you with available. Not all meaningful tasks require you to leave your house. But if the home is where you spend most your time hosting pity parties, then you would be better off selecting activities that are away from home.

Is there a hobby you once enjoyed? Find groups with the same interest and get to know them. While you're getting to know them, allow them to know you.

Doing something will break the chains unhappiness have tried to forge over your life. By doing something constructive, you train your brain to move your life toward a better outcome. By doing something, your emotions are forced into submission. By doing something, everyone you work with will be affected by the new you.

I learned the power of doing something while stuck in the biggest pity party ever. I was young; life had kicked me in the head. I had walked away from the principles taught to me I tried to cover myself-pity with a bottle the bottom of which exposed more unhappiness. I went to work every day, not for a paycheck, but to avoid other people.

One day I heard someone give a speech about attitude and action. I realized my attitude was leading me to the wrong actions, and my actions were promoting bad attitudes. I needed to break the cycle. Unfortunately, my attitude was so bad changing it first seemed impossible, so I changed my actions. I stopped hiding from people. I started getting involved with a church. Before I knew it, my attitude was starting to change in the right direction. As my attitude changed, I got more interested in other things. Bit-by-bit life took on a better outlook.

Did all my problems go away? No. Did new challenges show up? Yes. But, because I was active and my attitude was improving, the way I responded to the problems changed. By responding better, the outcomes became better. Did I solve every problem? No.

Why am I telling you this? You need to understand that being happy is not a cure-all. All your problems will not disappear overnight. Nor will the world forget everything you both said and did when unhappy. But your ability to go forward and get through life's challenges will be significantly improved.

These are the initial steps you need to change your course and head toward happiness. If you will apply these seven steps, not only will you start to see a change, others will see it as well.

Step number one: Choose to be happy
Step number two: Cultivate thanksgiving
Step number three: Practice forgiveness
Step number four: Counteract wrong thoughts and feelings
Step number five: Money will not make you happy
Step number six: Foster friendships
Step number seven: Engage in worthwhile activities.

eight
Health Issues

God, grant me the serenity to accept the things I cannot change,
Courage to change the things I can,
And wisdom to know the difference.
— Reinhold Niebuhr

Having health issues can cause lots of stress. This stress can, in turn, make it difficult to be happy. However, health issues do not make it impossible to be happy. Let me first make one thing clear. There is a big difference between being happy, having a positive outlook, and being in denial. Denial seeks to pretend the problem does not exist, while being happy and having the right perspective involve how you chose to handle the situation. How to handle your situation is the focus of this chapter.

In the summer of 2006, I was diagnosed with an end-stage renal disease. The situation required me to begin kidney dialysis. Dialysis is a three-day-a-week, four-hour treatment with no end date in sight, unless I get a transplant. Dialysis also required surgery to enable me to connect to the machine. The entire ordeal was disconcerting.

I was on an emotional trampoline. One moment I was fighting fear, the next I was in denial. Faced with a new set of doctors and procedures, I wanted to run away. To make matters worse, when I finally started on dialysis, all the patients in the unit looked like the unhappiest people in the world. It may be true that misery loves company, but misery is a poor hostess.

My first reaction to seeing the people and dealing with dialysis was to sequester myself at home. I did not want anyone to see me in such a poor state of body or mind. Well-meaning people tried to encourage me with horror stories of people they knew who had been on dialysis. When I would ask, "How was the person doing now?" without exception they would tell me the person was dead.

One day I was sitting next to an elderly lady, and she was smiling, at dialysis! I could not believe this woman. Maybe the woman was on drugs, or senile. I would not stop looking at her, and she would not stop smiling. Finally, she noticed me gaping and said, "I am so glad that dialysis is not my life".

Dialysis is what I do on the way to living my life. "Here was a lady much older than I, who had been on dialysis for years. But her outlook was unlike anyone's I had seen. For her dialysis was only a means to an end and not an end in itself. Because she looked at her situation differently, it empowered her to respond differently. The realization of what she said changed my life. I was still on dialysis. I was still having health issues with more to come, but now I had a new outlook. From that situation and others, I learned three things that enable me to be happy, even with health issues.

The first thing: When confronting health issues remain calm. I realize that when we get bad medical news, the mind wants to go into overdrive, but losing your peace will not help you deal correctly. As a matter of fact, by being calm, you may discover that the situation is not as bad as it seems. However, if it is bad, being calm will still enable you to process information better.

By remaining calm, you will be able to ask the right questions to get all the facts. You will need to do some research. Go online and get information that will help you understand your health issue. I made the mistake of listening to people who were well intentioned but lacked knowledge. I needed to investigate for myself. Getting more information helps bring reason and rationality to your situation.

Next, you will need to get as much support as you can. This includes family, friends, and support groups. By developing a support system, you override the temptation to isolate yourself. There is no shame in needing people or help. Many great support groups are more than willing to help you. The key is your willingness to open up and let people in. Do not allow fear to drive you into hiding. Once in it it will be hard to come out.

That brings us to the third point. Redirect your focus. Illness tries to drive our focus inward. When you are not feeling well, it is easy to focus only on your problems. But as stated in the Serenity Prayer, "Accept the things you cannot change." Acceptance is not resignation. Acceptance is acknowledging what is genuine and not getting stuck on that information, but moving forward.

Redirecting your focus will lessen the impact of your issues and lower any anxiety you may be having. It will amaze you just how much better you feel when your attention is off yourself. This is an excellent time to visit a friend who is having problems. Take time out to help them or get involved with a charity. Being truly happy is not about getting everything you want. It is, in part, about being grateful for what you already have. Sometimes we need to get involved helping others to appreciate what we do have.

Most importantly, look for the positive. No matter how bad things seem there is always something positive for you to focus on. I finally realized that even though I required dialysis I was still able to work every day. Take inventory of good people and things in your life. The key to being happy while dealing with health issues is not to allow your health to define you. You are not the total of your symptoms. At no stage of your fight to restore your health will your legal name be changed to the name of your disease. Instead of thinking about your limitation think about what you can do.

I found myself unable to travel without help. Being stuck in the house was a personal nightmare until I found something positive to do while at home. I started calling people who were trapped in the house and spent time encouraging them. I wanted to help them find ways to be positive about not being able to get out. You, too, can be a blessing to others as you win battles, and that will make you happy.

nine
Divorce

Every stage of life presents us with challenges, but very few can compare with divorce. Divorce or separation can hit you like a brick. It can take us on a trip you never planned on. One of the questions that echo through your whole being, "Will I ever be happy again?" This chapter takes into consideration that you have read the earlier seven steps in the book. The goal here is to address some of the things you need to consider if you are divorced.

First, it is ok to have different feelings; you are divorced. Divorce is the breakup of both physical and emotion bonds. Those bonds tied into every area of your life. Now you have to reorder your life without that person and while inundated with bad feelings. However, do not let those feelings lie to you. There is a few lies that will attempt to flood your thinking: One is that you were truly happy while married to your ex. The second lie is that you were always miserable. Both of these extremes are wrong. Over a period of time you were both of these, but not from beginning to end.

Give yourself permission to be upset, angry, or hurt. You have been through something, and it is not your fault the marriage did not work out. Because it takes two people to make a marriage, you were not in it by yourself. So, call your friends and cry, laugh or both, but do not think that drinking, drugs or some reckless act will make you feel better. If you are lucky being reckless will only make things worse.

Divorce brings about a sense of loss, second only to the loss experienced when someone dies. There are three areas of loss caused by a divorce; one is the loss of companionship. This is the one that rips at your heart. It produces the feeling of loneliness and tries to convince you that it is forever. This loss wants you to focus on your past. The second loss is that of support; financially, emotionally, and socially. This loss tries to make feel insecure. "How will I survive?" is the question you may be asking. This loss wants you to worry about the present. Then comes the third loss, the loss of hope and dreams. This loss is an attack on your view of the future.

Each of these losses is real but not permanent. They will last as long as you allow them to. Bear in mind that some things require time to recover. That is not a reason for them to remain forever. One thing you need to do is let go. Avoid talking about your ex all the time. Yes, you are hurt. Your pain is real, but as stated in an earlier chapter, wounds do not heal if you keep picking at them. As for support, you can and will rebound. You possess a greater ability to survive than you know. Your future is high as your imagination will envision it to be.

Now, take a break, it is time for you to take care of yourself. Money may be tight, but you need to do some things that will put you on the road to a better life. This process will require you to take care of yourself physically and emotionally. This self-care should include diet, exercise, and a makeover. Then join a support group. You need to see that others have been where you are and have made out just fine.

Understand one thing: you still have a future. To get to that future will entail hard work, but the rewards are worth it. Start toward your future by finding new activities. New activities will get you around new people and focus your thinking in new and creative ways. If you have children find new things you can do together. There were things you were interested in besides being married, explore some of those interests. Do not define yourself as somebody's ex-spouse; redefine yourself. Take that class, start the business, write that book, or take that vacation. You have a new set of options. Use them.

Moving forward is your goal, but if you have children they need to come with you. To bring them along you must minimize the impact of the situation on your kids. Here is how you do it:

- Reassure and listen to your children.
- Maintain stability.
- Provide consistent discipline and instruction.
- Let your kids know they can rely on you.
- Do not assume they know how you feel about them, tell them.
- Do not put your children in your conflict with their other parent.
- Tell them every day that together we can make it.

Lastly, you have to think positively. You have plenty to offer the world, and it is time to show it off. Remember, do not let your situation define you. It is your life and your dictionary; define yourself, and make it a magnificent definition. In time life will get back to normal. Just realize it will be a new normal. Decide that the new normal will be a better one. Be happy.

ten
Grief

Although there are predictable and universal aspects of grieving, each person's experience is unique. The phases and their tasks are most often described in chronological sequence, but in reality, they assume a "hop-scotch" sequence: individuals may proceed through two or three phases only to find themselves back to "start" some six months later.

We have come to the subject of grief. Please keep in mind the steps presented in chapters one through seven as we address this issue. The intensity of pain that grief causes will lessen, but the sense of that grief comes and goes, for seemingly no reason, often for years.

On Monday March 3, 1969, at 12:20 pm, my maternal grandfather passed away. Although I was only ten years old, I was very close to him. All the adults attempted to console me, but with little success. By the time his memorial services were over, I thought everything would be ok. However, two years later while sitting in seventh grade science class, I started crying. Tears just started flowing. My teacher asked me to step out into the hallway. He wanted to know what was going on? I told him, "My grandfather died." Remember, no one had a cell phone.

So he asked me," When did your grandfather die?"

"Two years ago" I replied.

Without warning, I had remembered it was March 3rd, again, and the tears started and would not stop.

My goal, in this chapter, is not to help you get over your grief but to get through it. This book is not a counseling manual. Please seek the help of a therapist, or minister for help. This chapter will aid in your recovery, but is no substitute for grief counseling.

When dealing with grief, there have been many models developed to explain the process. These models were not designed to minimize the reality of loss, but to provide a tool to empower others to understand and help those who are grieving. I have included this chapter because, in your quest for happiness, there will be life events that derail that desire.

Grief stops the flow of your routine, brings forward momentum to a halt. Understanding how to work your way through this pain provides light at the end of a seemingly endless dark tunnel.

In dealing with grief, I prefer the approach used by Dr. Susan J. Zonnebelt-Smeenge and Dr. Robert C. DeVries. They talk about the things you need to accomplish to move through the process of grief to go forward into your new life. Grief as H.N. Wright says:

" is an individual journey, yet there are the five specific tasks with corresponding behaviors that you need to address to help you move through your grief detour."

The order of this process is not important, but each part is essential.

First, you need to come to grips with the reality of the loss. The person you cared about has died and is unable to return. And if you believed the Bible and the person did, too, they would not want to return. Emotionally accepting this fact is the greatest obstacle you can overcome.

Second, you need to express all of your feelings regarding this matter.

She Died From Suppressed Grief

Dr. Erick Linderman, psychiatrist-in-chief of the Massachusetts General Hospital and a pioneer in the investigation of repressed sorrow, tells of a young nurse who tended her father through the long winter of his final illness. She was very devoted to her father, and often fought back tears as she nursed him.

When he died, a well-meaning friend sternly forbade her to show any grief for the sake of her mother who had a weak heart. Within hours, the emotionally-repressed nurse developed a case of ulcerate colities. She slowly corroded inwardly because of her nervous system. Eventually she died, killed by the suppressed grief she would not allow herself to express in copious tears. — Ministers' Research Service

Holding in the pain you feel will only prolong your recovery and could make matters worse. I realize that for the sake of other family members you have to be strong, and maybe even handle the last affairs of that loved one. But at some point, even if alone, you need to express how you feel. Again, seek professional help.

Third, H.N. Wright says," You need to sort through and identify the memories of your loved one, and find a place to store them so you can begin to move on. This task basically means that because your loved one is no longer present--no longer a dynamic and active part of your ongoing journey--you need to make him or her a vital and rich memory of your life".

This step prepares you for all that follows and prevents you from taking up residence in a permanent state of grief. It will enable you to move beyond any anger or guilt you needed to address in step two. Again, grief is a normal part of life; the goal is not to allow the pain to become your whole life.

Fourth, recognize who you are apart from your departed loved one. If it was your last living parent, are you now an orphan? If your spouse, are you still married? Or single? Or would you call yourself widowed? Reevaluating your identity is a vital component of your grief recovery.

Lastly, getting through grief requires that you invest in the life you have going forward. What are your personal interests, desires, and dreams from this new perspective? What lifestyle changes will you make? How will you reconfigure your priorities?

The journey forward will be what you chose to make it. Remember you are stronger, smarter and more gifted than you realize. You will survive and thrive. Why? Because you chose to.

eleven

Suicide

*"There is a way that seemeth right unto a man, but the end thereof
are the ways of death."*

Proverbs 14:12 (King James Version)

According to the Center for Disease Control (CDC) suicide is the
tenth leading cause of death in the United States for all ages. The
number of suicides is a key indication of the overall level of unhappiness in which so many people find themselves. A key factor in produc-
ing this state of sadness is the proliferation of bad news. Twenty-four
hours a day through television, radio, and the Internet bad news is
freely dispensed. News regarding politics, the economy, our schools,
the environment, and police shootings fill our ears and minds with an
abundance of concerns. Every day special interest groups proclaim
a plethora of disasters on the horizon. All of the bad news is com-
pounded by the personal issues we face in day-to-day living. Without
a conscious effort to counteract all the bad news surrounding us being
happy is an uphill battle.

Suicide will not make you happy, nor is it the fix for unhappiness.
At best, suicide is a permanent decision in a failed attempt to fix a temporary problem. Suicide is based on the belief that quitting is the only
option, but the truth is that quitting is never the right answer, and once

completed, cannot be undone. But for a person to get to this point he/she must believe several lies, and they must think that all hope is gone. The desire to commit suicide can come about when someone is depressed, ashamed, deeply hurt or in despair. But all of these situations are temporary, and everyone has the power to overcome the situations that life can bring.

A person must believe that suicide will solve their problems. This lie assumes that in death there are no issues, but what if you are wrong and instead of getting away from one problem you go to a bigger problem? To make matters worst you cannot undo what you have done. The old adage "Where there is life there is hope" is true. As long as you live, things can and will change.

Do not believe the lie that if you die all of your issues will be solved.

Some believe there is nothing after death. However, interviews with patients who were declared clinically dead and then brought back are clear that death is just the beginning. Unfortunately, not everyone has reported a pleasant experience; some have come back screaming.

Death is not the end.

You have plenty to offer; God has made you of great value. The pressures of life present you opportunities to demonstrate your God-given ability to overcome any and everything life brings. However, many times the key to victory rests in a willingness to ask for help. You have more to live for than your present situation may reveal, so do not believe the lie that there is no need to continue living. History has proven that even the most isolated person impacts others. As a matter of fact, on average no less than seven people are affected.

The thief comes only in order to steal and kill and destroy. I came that they may have and enjoy life, and have it in abundance [to the full, till it overflows].

John 10:10 Amplified Bible (AMP)

Noun Suicide
1. the intentional taking of one's own life.

The desire to commit suicide is the highest expression of unhappiness. The events that bring people to this point are numerous and beyond the scope of this book. Persons contemplating suicide should seek professional help. The aim of this chapter is to provide some options for consideration.

Throughout this book I have presented key steps to regaining lasting Happiness. If you have skipped to this chapter, I recommend that you take the time to start from the beginning of the book and apply its teachings to your life. Hopefully, by the time you return to this chapter, it will not be needed.

"For God so [greatly] loved and dearly prized the world, that He [even] gave His [One and only begotten] Son, so that whoever believes and trusts in Him [as Savior] shall not perish, but have eternal life. John 3:16 Amplified Bible (AMP)

Hear my cry, O God; attend unto my prayer. From the end of the earth will I cry unto thee, when my heart is overwhelmed: lead me to the rock that is higher than I. Psalm 61:1-2 KJV

Being overwhelmed by the issues of life is something that affects everyone sooner or later. There is no shame in being overwhelmed, nor in realizing that you cannot make things better on your own. Coming to the end of yourself is the first step to getting the answers and the help you need. It is when you can go no farther that your heart, broken though it may be, is ready to receive what God has to offer. God is that Rock that will lift you above everything you are dealing with, and He will give you real peace.

For God so loved the world, that he gave his only begotten Son,

that whosoever believeth in him should not perish, but have everlasting life.
John 3:16 KJV

Your life is precious to God. Life is God's gift to you and how you use that life is an expression of your appreciation for the gift. Many times life falls apart because we have not honored God who blessed us with life, and we have done everything contrary to His plans for us. But the good news is that it is not too late, and that is why you are reading this book. God is reaching out to you to tell you that He knew this day would come and had this chapter added to this book just for you. This book was finished and ready for publication, but God would not let it be published until this chapter was added.

Regardless of how it looks, God loves you and only wants the best for you. He sent Jesus to die on the cross to pay the debt sin caused. Your way is not working but God has a better way, and it begins with your surrendering your life to Him. You do not have to carry the hurt, pain, grief, sorrow, or despair anymore. He wants to take it off your hands. That is why He sent Jesus to die for your sins, so that God could carry the load for you. If your heart is overwhelmed, it is time to cry out to God.

Pray this prayer:

God, I admit that my way is not working. I bring to you my life with all its problems. I confess that I have sinned and not honored you who have given me life. I ask that through the work that Jesus did on the cross you forgive me, and I accept Jesus as your answer for my problem and as Lord of my life.

Amen.

twelve
The End and The Beginning

We have come to the end of this book, but the beginning of your journey. Through the pages of this book we have given seven steps:

1. Choose to be happy, regardless
2. Cultivate thanksgiving
3. Practice forgiveness
4. Counteract thoughts and feelings
5. Money will not make you happy
6. Foster friendships
7. Engage in worthwhile activities

Briefly we address:
- Health issues
- Divorce
- Grief

Refer to this book often. Re-read the chapters that speak to your situation, and give it time to help you make changes in your life. It is my hope that this book was able to help you. If you know someone who could use

46

this book, buy them a copy. Your buying someone a copy of this book, would be an excellent way to invest into another's life.

Share the things you have learned with as many people as you can. By sharing with others in this way, you will reinforce the facts with-in yourself. Develop a sense of purpose, not only to be happy, but to see those around you happy as well.

Get up every morning determined to win the battles life will present you. Win these battles by starting your day with declarative statements.

- "I will be happy today."
- "I will face today ready for whatever life brings."
- "All of my life experiences have groomed me for today."
- "With God's help this day will end with me on top."
- "I will take a moment to help others get through this day."
- "I will seek out those who are struggling and provide aid."

By starting your days with these declarations, you will tap into the source of happiness that only comes to people who dare step outside the box. Give this process of daily declarations thirty days. Keep a journal during this period to track your moods, people you help, and things you accomplish.

At the end of the thirty days review your journal. Use what you have learned to add to or modify your declarative statements. If you are impressed, you can share the outcome with friends what you have done and encourage them to give it a try.

Get Your Free Workbook: http://bit.ly/2jKjibN

Please feel free to contact me with any questions you have regarding the steps in this book. Email: *Behappy@jamesewoods.net* Please enter "be happy" in the subject line.

Visit my blog: http://bit.ly/2jyfKwa
Connect on Facebook: http://bit.ly/2jArjTd
I look forward to hearing from you.

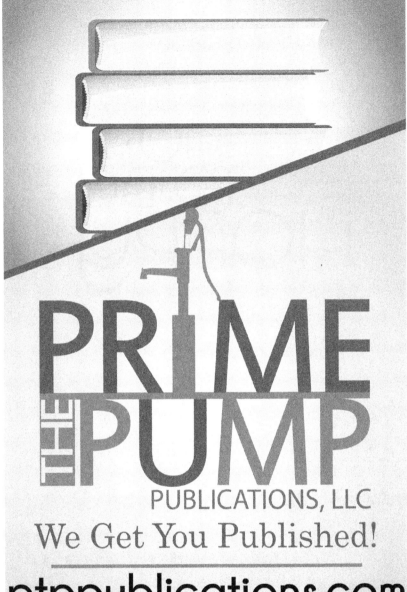

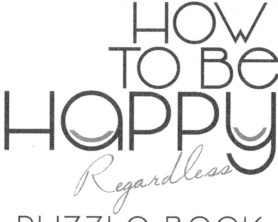

HOW TO BE HAPPY Regardless

PUZZLE BOOK

BY
JAMES E. WOODS

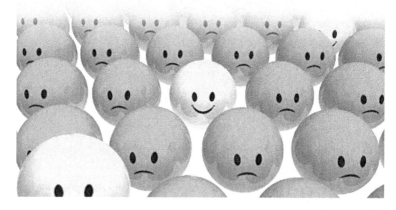

CPSIA information can be obtained
at www.ICGtesting.com
Printed in the USA
BVOW03*1145150517
483242BV00018B/17/P